I0412502

There *IS* no Stage 5

(blessed with cancer)

Linda Parrish

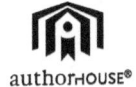

authorHOUSE®

AuthorHouse™
1663 Liberty Drive
Bloomington, IN 47403
www.authorhouse.com
Phone: 1-800-839-8640

First published by AuthorHouse 7/15/2011

ISBN: 978-1-4634-2326-1 (sc)
ISBN: 978-1-4634-2325-4 (e)

Printed in the United States of America

Any people depicted in stock imagery provided by Thinkstock are models,
and such images are being used for illustrative purposes only.
Certain stock imagery © Thinkstock.

This book is printed on acid-free paper.

Dedicated to:

My husband, Larry– who is my rock.
My daughter, Angela– who is my joy.
My sisters Marilyn, Karen and Janice – for their unconditional love and support.
My parents – who raised me right.

A special thanks to the oncologists at KU Med Center for saving my life.

It started out like any ordinary life; at least *I* thought so. I figured every kid on my block and in my school was just like me. You know, happily married parents, siblings, pets, church on Sunday in matching outfits their mom made, followed by the much anticipated trip to McDonalds…stuff like that. Life was so simple in the mid '50s in New York.

Spending the first eight years of my youth on Long Island in the perfect neighborhood, with my perfect family, again seemed ordinary. I was unaware of ugly things like divorce, adultery, sexual abuse, cussing, alcohol, drugs, and cancer. I knew about broken bones, stitches, the flu, mercurochrome, and Band-Aids. That's about as bad as it ever got.

My early childhood was right out of Pleasantville. No worries, played all the time, had some chores and dinner with the family every night. Rarely was it from a restaurant; maybe pizza once in awhile. The

Wonderful World of Disney Saturday nights and Ed Sullivan on Sunday as the six of us gathered around our small black & white television set. We had a half acre of woods behind us; great for exploring, making forts and climbing trees. We looked for arrowheads to make spears and conquer "the enemy." Marilyn and I developed our own language which was fun to use around friends or sisters if we wanted to share secrets (Still do it to this day!). I must say, living in the last house on a dead-end street was awesome. It was very conducive for dodge ball, four-square, red light/green light and various other games played with the neighborhood gang.

Next to us was an abandoned sump surrounded by a 20-foot fence and gate. The city would open it up in winter so we could ride our sleds down the huge, sloped sides. Of course a locked fence did not stop us from digging underneath it to enter that treasure pit of the unknown, anytime we pleased. There were enormous round rocks (geodes) we would crack open using smaller rocks as hammers that would unveil a most glorious center. Filled with crystals, mica, quartz, and beautiful prismatic colors, our little eyes flew wide open in amazement! Most days were spent on our bikes, often carrying a stuffed animal in the basket on the handlebars. Sometimes we even put one of our cats or the dog in doll clothes and pushed them around in a baby stroller. You know they had to love *that*. We would be gone from after breakfast till dinnertime, never checking in with Mom. Can you imagine that happening today?

On the other side of the sump, the city planted huge potato fields that went all the way to the highway that took you to the city. There were areas that dipped low in the ground, so when it rained, scattered ponds were formed in the fields. In winter these ponds became skating rinks. Since we lived the closest, we would put on our single blade skates with rubber covers, and trek about 20 minutes over the frozen bumpy ground to the biggest pond. We would skate for hours, being careful not to go too close to the thin ice areas. Once our friend Jeff fell through and we had to carry his ice-soaked, limp body back to our house. Mom had hot cocoa with marshmallows ready for us (Made from scratch. Didn't have instant back then). We put our wet clothes on the radiator to dry then wrapped up in a blanket and got all toasty. Often we hunkered down on the couch to watch *Howdy Doody*. Marilyn and I were on that show once. What a hoot! We sat in the "Peanut Gallery." Any of you remember that? She kept elbowing me, telling me not to pick my nose. I did it anyway just to make her mad, not thinking that the kids at school would see me on TV and give me grief for days. Idiot! I was always doing something where she had to rescue me or get me out of trouble. Being a tomboy, she would often beat up the neighborhood bully when he got out of control. Andy Cabott. Some names you never forget.

Even though I had three sisters and many friends, I created an imaginary pal for awhile. She never sassed me or said she didn't want to play what I wanted. Eventually that bored me, so I made a ghost from one of Dad's handkerchiefs, drew on a face and tied a string around its neck. I pretended it was flying over my head everywhere I went, when it was really being dragged along the ground. Guess I had to invent a lot of things to occupy my free time.

Kids today have no clue how great life was back then. No computers, no cell phones, no video games or iPods. We just rode our bikes, roller-skated or played with board games, cards, jump rope, Barbies, GI Joes, or army guys. So simple. So easy.

I loved New York for the incredible seasons. When it was winter...*it was winter!* Not only did we have the ponds to skate on, but there were big hills full of deep snow for sledding. One of our friends lived way up on this hill and every winter they would open up their snow-filled, hilly yard and driveway to all the kids. The driveway was long and curvy, so when we reached the bottom on our sleds, we would crash into a snow bank to avoid going into the busy street. Then the dad would come down on a tractor with a flatbed so we could all climb on the back, dragging our sleds, and travel the long way back up to do it again...and again. For a change of pace, we would sled or ski down the wavy slopes in their huge yard and try not to slide under the fence at the bottom and into the street.

Living close enough to water, we experienced many hurricanes. We would look out our large windows to see trees, lawn furniture, trash, and rocks fly by. One time someone's doghouse went sailing past. We often feared something would crash through the glass and kill us. It was really cool!

Summertime meant Jones Beach and Coney Island. Too much fun! Sand in your britches for days, carnival rides and cotton candy till you puked. Fall was so beautiful since we were surrounded by huge trees, not to mention that half acre of woods. Springtime was awesome as well. We often went to the zoo and these great parks to feed the ducks. It was a perfect childhood.

In the early '60s Dad got a promotion so we moved to Kansas City, where I *totally* did not fit in. Picture this - starting out in the 4th grade at a new school, in a new state, in a new frilly dress with a horrible haircut. "The Pixie" - basically a short, boyish hairdo with stupid long sideburns. Just awful! To make bad matters worse, I was a chubby kid who talked 100 miles a minute. (New Yorker, remember?) These Midwesterners d-r-a-w-l-e-d out their words and made me crazy! No one liked me; and even ran from me on the playground screaming as if I were a monster (well...that was after I blurted out in the lunchroom, "I HATE Kansas City. Kansas City

STINKS!!!"). They were all making fun of my accent, so I had to say *something*, right?

As if we did not stand out enough, one day Marilyn and I wore our "Beatle" wigs to school. They were actually stupid fuzzy hats in white (the one I wore) and black (hers). What were we thinking? They didn't resemble **real** hair let alone a Beatle 'do! Odder still, it was summer, so sweat poured down our faces. But we were COOL, right? What a couple of dorky kids.

Our eldest sister, Karen, was your basic drama queen when we were growing up. She would often sing and act in her bedroom. Marilyn and I would sneak in there, go under her bed and giggle. One time we lay down and pulled the curtains slowly back and forth to scare her while she was in one of her acting modes in front of the mirror. She took off shrieking. It was great punking her. Janice, on the other hand, was the baby and stole all the focus from me when she came along. I was the baby for 7 years and loved it! All of a sudden, here is this new kid in the house that everyone is slobbering over. I would do everything in my power to draw all eyes and ears to me. Had to be the center of attention. (funny… that hasn't changed). I remember terrorizing her and throwing her around, often resulting in her smashing into a wall or something. She would cry out for Mom, and I would beg her to calm down or try to bribe her not to tell on me. Never worked. I got spanked; which made me want to beat her up even more. Sibling jealousy is an ugly animal (Kinda cool that we are extremely close now, though).

Another great memory was making popcorn balls with Mom. There was a large pass-through opening from the family room to the kitchen. I would pull up a kitchen chair, sit on my knees and lean through the opening to reach the counter. Mom would make popcorn in a big pan, then boil Karo syrup and slowly pour it over the popcorn. She had me butter my hands so I could roll up the hot popcorn into balls. We didn't know then that butter was the worst thing you could put on your skin when handling hot foods. After they were formed into somewhat spherical little orbs, I covered them in Saran Wrap and tied the ends with curly ribbon. These would be given out at Halloween, or just for us to enjoy.

At Christmastime, we made something really neat for guests that visited. We cracked open walnuts, scooped out the nuts (to be used in cookies later) then placed a tiny trinket in the shell. The two halves were held together with a red velvet ribbon with a loop added at the top. We made about 12 or so and attached them on a long strip of ribbon and hung it on the back of the front door. There was a bell at the bottom that would gently ring when the door was opened. When the guests would leave, they got to choose a prize from the ribbon. Everyone loved it!

Mom was the queen of holiday cookies. The variety ranged from oatmeal crisps, spritzes, Swedish rosettes, rum balls, and decorated sugar cookies that we made with cookie cutters shaped in trees, snowmen, Santas, and candy canes. Everyone loved exchanging cookies with our family. Good times.

During my "teenage angst" years that followed, I always thought I was blessed, or led a sort of charmed life. I believed God existed, but took my sweet time becoming a true "believer" by asking Jesus into my life. I was having WAY too much fun partying! I thought if I became a Christian, I would never have fun again my entire life. I could never sin...never drink, swear, smoke, dance, date boys...whatever, because I had "given in" and asked Him to be my Savior. So it was quite awhile before I ever entertained that thought again. After all, **I** was the one putting on eye makeup during the sermon or passing notes to my friends when everyone else was praying. I already *knew* I was going to Hell!!

Then there was my bout with shoplifting. My older friend Kim and I would ride our bikes to the local shopping center--your basic square, brick building with about 20 shops around the perimeter, a bowling alley to the left of it and a gas station to the right. We entered the Pinkie's Ben Franklin and dead-headed it to the "penny aisle." There were wooden trays filled with a zillion knickknacks, doo-bobs...you know, stuff used for crafts. Since there were no cameras or curvy mirrors and people were more trusting, we had no trouble loading our pockets full of these tiny gems. Let's not forget the "penny candy" section! We always bought something so the cashiers would think we were truly shopping, as they were unaware that the bulges in our clothes were due to the many things we were NOT buying! Back on our bikes, we rode to the ladies' room in the gas station where there was a long pink tile vanity for us to display our loot. After looking over our separate piles, we kept or traded our favorites. Here's the crazy part. We then rode back to the store and returned the items we did *not* want, never thinking that we could just as easily get busted putting things back! Dumb kids.

Eventually we got bored with that caper and wanted to go bigger: the grocery store. Our plan was to go to the candy bar aisle, one of us taking a huge chocolate bar and calling out to the other, "You think Mom would let us get this?" Whoever had the candy would hold it up repeating that question as if we were actually looking for our mom. We figured shoppers and clerks would see and hear us and think it was all real. We'd locate an empty aisle and shove it in a pocket or under our shirt. It worked once for her, but when it was my turn, I got stopped at the exit. I looked up to see the head checker who was also my mom's Avon lady. I wanted to die. Everyone was staring at me as she loudly reprimanded me and threatened to tell my parents. I sheepishly handed her the candy as my friend ran off. That episode scared me straight and kept me from a possible life of crime (Well…who knows?).

I had gotten myself into trouble many times in my late teens, but somehow always managed to pull out of it before anything major happened. I was a party girl, stayed out late, lied to my folks, and always felt bad about it; because they were the perfect parents, remember? Pleasantville? In my heart, I knew God was making things OK for me. I just knew He was watching over me and not allowing me to go too far. I just didn't know why I was special enough to receive His blessings. I certainly did not feel I deserved any.

In high school I was accepted in all cliques, as there was not one for people like me – whatever that means. I had friends in the jocks, the nerds, the 2%ers, the freaks, the choir, the band, the artsy-fartsy's, and whoever was left. I was funny, so all types of people liked me, I guess. If there was some prank to pull, they would count on me to be a big part of it. I think I depended on my sense of humor to get me places and to hopefully be popular. Sadly, it only landed me in the principal's office on a regular basis.

I knew I wasn't the scholarly type, so when I graduated, I only wanted to work and make lots of money (Like two or three part-time jobs selling shoes would get me there). Six months of that, and I decided community college would be better, especially since my two best friends went there. I had no idea what I wanted to do with my life, career wise, so I partied most of the time in-between classes. I truly do not know how I made it through, as I was pretty blurry most of the day. After my true love dumped me, I got more serious about my future. I went two more years to another local community college to study Animal

Health Technology. I practiced for about 10 months, and knew it was not for me. Back to sales I went. This is what I knew. This is what I was good at.

Fast forward to the late '70s. I was selling wholesale liquor (go figure) and met and dated a chef I sold to. I thought that was it. I had dated a lot of losers and felt I was approaching the spinster age, so figured I'd better get hitched – quickly! We ended up dating, lived together four years, finally married, had a daughter, and then divorced. Eleven years with the wrong guy. He was unfaithful from day one. I did not see it, or maybe chose NOT to see it. I was a good wife and homemaker, a good mother, had a great job, and balanced everything perfectly – in my mind anyway. So why would he want to be with someone else if I was so great? I had a difficult time accepting this failure, and the stigma of being a divorcée and a single mother. I also had to endure the loss and emptiness of a miscarriage about a year before I got pregnant with Angela. At that time I thought I would never have the daughter I always wanted. I conceived on my 32nd birthday. She was born in '86. I divorced him in '88.

While living in my beautiful 50-year-old Tudor home, filled with antiques, a 2-year old, and a dog, I thought about dating again. Not only was I searching for someone for me, but he had to be the right fit to be an instant father – if we ended up getting married that is. No one was really up to my standards, but I kept looking. I did not like being on my own. I did not like being lonely.

I was helping my mom teach Sunday school at the church I grew up in. I enjoyed the time together; plus the 4-year olds were a riot. I had been doing this for about a year before I got pregnant, and returned when Angela was a few months old. It felt good to be back and doing something positive for others, plus kids that age are just funny. They speak the truth and don't care what you think about it. Art Linkletter was right, huh? Kids DO say the darndest things! I kept this up till the early '90s when Mom retired.

The minister was the neatest guy I had ever met. He was nice looking, and had a voice that purred at the pulpit. You couldn't help but savor every word. When I was a kid, he would hang out with the youth, tell great stories, and do handstands and flips. We all thought he was the coolest! I am trying to remember the exact time and place that I finally became a Christian. I know it was years before all this happened. Funny...most people would note this as a most significant part of their life, but I just accepted it as a natural thing to do.

Other than a wrecked marriage, I had more unsettling things happen to me that I eventually bounced back from. On the way to a mandatory 6 a.m. Saturday inventory, my life would change suddenly. Barefoot and seat beltless, I dead-headed it to work. No one was allowed to miss this inventory crap unless you died, or were close to it! Well, I would soon fit that bill. Who is on neighborhood streets at that hour on a Saturday? It was some young girl, possibly on her way back from a party, trying to make it home before her parents woke up. She apparently didn't see the flashing red light; since she blew right threw it. While driving slowly through the yellow flashing light, I saw a blur of color to the right of me. The next thing I knew I was slowly opening my eyes and looking out my passenger side window – my chin resting on the glassless opening. Strangely enough, both knees were on the floor on *my* side of the car, so my body was all pretzeled up.

I realized I was alive because I could feel the intense pain on my left side. Minutes later, there were firemen and policemen with the "jaws of life" trying to figure out how to pry me from my crumpled car. All I could think to do was to ask everyone for a phone to call my boss. I did NOT want to get fired for not showing up for that blasted inventory. Can you tell I pretty much hated it? I usually got stuck in the cooler or up on the forklifts counting pallets of dog food or something exciting (I was a sales gal, NOT a warehouse guy!). I cracked jokes with the ambulance people, but they had no sense of humor. I told them what to do about all my belongings and of course, to get me a damn phone. I still can't believe I was more worried about being missed at work than my own well being. Did I mention that when the girl hit me, my car careened 40 feet across a parking lot and smacked into a brick wall? That was the last thing

I saw before I heard a voice say, or maybe *I* said out loud, "I'm dead!"

The emergency room doctor was mystified as to why my knee was not shattered in a million pieces. The force of it slamming into the dash broke the dashboard in half. The heat from the impact melted the vinyl of the dash onto my pants. He kept taking more x-rays but my knee was fine. However, I did have three broken ribs on the left side – snapped clean in two. The rest of me resembled a battered wife poster, complete with black eyes, lumps, and bruises in all colors. But...I survived! It was as if a huge hand came down from the sky and grabbed my head to pull me back – like it was some Heavenly message sent to me saying "Not now, Linda." By the way, that brick wall I hit was a church.

10 weeks of recovery and I was good as new.

While resting upstairs one afternoon, my daughter (now 4) was playing outside with the girl next door. Hours later her mom came over in a panic, asking me if my daughter mentioned the truck and the bad men. I looked down at her little face and asked her what the lady was talking about. She then began the telling of a most disturbing tale. She had a great knack for details, so it was akin to listening to a police report. These two creepy guys drove up slowly in a blue truck with the bed full of Little Tykes toys: a playhouse, a trike, stuff like that. The driver got out, left the door open, and approached the girls who were sitting at the curb playing. Neither of us moms knew that was going on, as they were *not* allowed to play near the street! Each of them told us they would be at the other one's house, that way they could do whatever they wanted (They start so young, don't they?).

The creepy guy became creepier. He asked them if they wanted to go for a ride in his truck, and that he had a duck in his pants if they wanted to pet it. Fortunately my baby girl had some *stranger danger* training in day care, and knew enough to grab her friend's hand and run away. The unfortunate part is they never told us till several hours had passed. We filed a police report, advised all the neighbors and kept a lookout for weeks. Along with *those* sleezeballs, our neighborhood was being "shopped" by nearby gangs or crack heads. My car was broken into twice, and the house was once while I was asleep. I *had* to move…west. The best schools were in Johnson County, Kansas, so that's where I looked. Wonder if that big hand came down again and pulled my little one away from danger? Or was every "close call" just a coincidence?

Lenexa, Kansas, offered the perfect home, in the perfect neighborhood, with the perfect backyard. This is where we would now be safe and I could start my life over. It was 1991, and I was no spring chicken. It had been close to a year since I had any real male companionship. The car wreck, recovery and the move kept me pretty occupied. I had a few dates since the divorce, but no big deal. My friends kept telling me that I was trying too hard. If I would just relax and concentrate on myself and not focus on getting a guy, the right one would come along. I had no idea what they were talking about and pretty much blew them off. What did *they* know? They weren't in my shoes!

With Angela attending kindergarten, decorating a four-bedroom home and working full time, I realized I actually *was* focusing on me…like what my friends were saying. I was so grateful to be alive and for having my daughter safe, that my priorities changed. I truly looked at the same things in a different way. I often pondered on the idea of praying about finding my Mr. Right. I thought that would be pretentious and pretty selfish, but I did it anyway. For the next two weeks I recited the same little prayer…always thanking God for saving my life and saying how grateful I was to be here and for all the blessings I felt I did not deserve. Then I would say, "If you have someone picked out for me…I think I am ready now."

At the end of two weeks of constant repetitive prayer, I had an awesome dream! I was on a plane coming back from some tropical place with my sister and I was in the aisle seat. I looked to my right and across from me sat this handsome man with dark hair with a touch of gray at the temples. Very distinguished looking. He had a dark moustache, deep, dark eyes, and (as a bonus) appeared to have a great build. He leaned towards me and said. "I can't wait to get back to Kansas City…well…Lenexa, actually." I replied, "I just moved to Lenexa, where do you live?" He said the name of my neighborhood. My eyes widened, my heart pounded, and I asked what his street address was, that maybe we were neighbors. He rambled off *my* address, and that he lived there with his wife, Linda, and step daughter, Angela. I got flushed and upset and stuttered, "That...that's me, and m-m-my address, my daughter, and I don't know who the Hell you are!" He turned to me, held my hands across the aisle, and looked into my eyes. A euphoric fog seemed to drift throughout the plane. He said. "I am your future. I am just here to tell you that everything is going to be alright. We will meet and fall in love, get married, and live in your house. But don't look for me. When you get off this plane, you will forget all about this, but do not worry." At this time, I turned to Janice and yelled "This guy just said, '*blah, blah, blah*'" then turned back around to see me holding the hands of some old fart instead. I jumped up from my seat, ran up and down the aisle, and then BAM... woke up in a cold sweat!

I spent the next several hours that day looking for "him" everywhere I went. Then I reminded myself that he said NOT to look for him. So I figured it was just sort of an omen of good things to come one day, and went on about my business. The next evening, I was all decked out ready to meet up with a friend for dinner. I had some time to kill. It was November 15, 1991, so I decided to go Christmas shopping at a nearby mall. While walking around aimlessly with no man to shop for, I looked up...and standing in front of a men's store was THE GUY FROM MY DREAM! I stopped in my tracks and even stopped breathing a little. What was I to do now? That was him – head to toe. A strong magnetism drew me to him, and seconds later we were talking like high schoolers. The flirting was over the top, but I didn't care. This was literally the man of my dreams, and I was *not* leaving!

We made plans to meet up later that night, but it didn't work out. I went out of town that weekend all aglow because I met "him." To my great surprise, he called Monday, we met up, and have been together ever since. We truly are soul mates, if that is a real thing; but it was not all wine and roses along the way. Many things we experienced as a couple could have destroyed our relationship, but I knew in my heart he was sent to me, so I was patient. Things would go up and down, good and bad for quite some time. Having the belief that God played a huge part in bringing us together kept me settled knowing everything would be ok, just like in my dream – which, by the way, was actually a vision. Larry and I were married in November of 1993. Everything happened just like in the dream.

In '94 I had my tubes tied. I was having some severe issues of the female nature. I wanted so badly to bear him a son, but I was also a bit long in the tooth, and may have had more problems than I wanted to take on. Then came the weight! It was as if the flood gates opened and no matter what I ate or drank, it went straight to my everywhere! I was no longer the blushing bride. More like the bulging cow. After that...rheumatoid arthritis. I woke one day to a totally stiff body, with fat, puffy feet, and hands like hooves. I could do nothing with my extremities! What happened?? My doctor said to take some water pills, as I must have been on a salt lick (Which I thought was possible since I had a margarita, potato chips, a dill pickle, and a Reuben the day before). Three days passed and I still could not *see* my feet, let alone put shoes on them! A blood test, a diagnosis, some pills, some pain, and my world continued. Great! Now I'm fat AND gimped up.

About this time I am thinking that my husband had to be thinking, "This is not what I bargained for. Where did my sexy wife go? Now I am stuck with this crippled-up chubster. No fair." I had no idea how much he really loved me until much later. My insecurity was all in my head.

We trudged onward in our relationship having the ordinary problems: money, disagreements, child rearing...oh, did I mention money? Then we started going to church as a family. That was really nice for all of us, until the church decided to fire the pastor, and all Hell broke loose. Some people stayed there with the "bad people" that fired him, some went to services elsewhere, but eventually the whole church family was divided. This hypocrisy sent my husband back to never going to church again. And he hasn't since. Raised in a strict fundamental Pentecostal church, with a military cop as his father, in a poor southern town, he had no normal childhood; only church-related activities. With no siblings, and the nearest kid miles away, he spent his free time reading. With all the tent revivals, foot washings, speaking in tongues, hands-on healings, and Jericho marches, he grew up despising church and religion in general. You can imagine that after finally coming back to church as an adult with his new family, then having that all torn apart… he was probably gone for good. I can't say that I blamed him, either.

If anything could shake a person's faith, this next series of events could do it. My dad and I were the best buddies. When I was in school in the late '70s for Animal Health Technology, Dad had a farm. I would go with him in his antique Studebaker truck to pill and work the cows. I even went with him on a three-hour trip to pick out our bull. I named him Bud. I was the only one of his four daughters that followed in his salesman footsteps. I started selling retail in high school, and then went on to outside sales/wholesale products. We would always compare sales tales and laugh. I was at his house every week to call in orders, and maybe have lunch as Mom would fix up something nutritionally good. I called him every night, too. We were very close.

In April of 1999, Mom was struggling with memory loss and repeating herself. Easter was right around the corner, and Dad called each of us crying to say she had just been diagnosed with Alzheimer's. He was planning to tell her on Easter Sunday with all the family there to help with her reaction. The unthinkable happened instead. He had a heart attack on Good Friday while sitting in his recliner. I was working in my garden when I got the call. I didn't even recognize my own mother's voice. The fact that she knew enough to remember my number was remarkable in itself.

She was hysterically crying while attempting to tell me, "I think your father is dead! He's not breathing! I can't get him to wake up!" I dropped the phone, jumped into my car and sped off towards her house. My eyes were so flooded with tears I could barely see, and was going about 90. I left my sleeping husband upstairs and flew by my daughter who was playing down the street. There was no time to explain. I called my three sisters, but could not reach any of them. I was going to have to face this alone.

I called 911, and they were there when I arrived. The paramedics would not let me see my dad, as they were on his chest trying to revive him. They wheeled him past me on the gurney and into the ambulance. I knew by looking at him he was gone. I had to stop my horrific pain so I could take care of my mom, who was in and out of awareness of the whole situation. She and I followed Dad to the hospital. By this time, I had reached my husband and daughter, who then came to meet us there. Still no sisters. This was NOT happening! My dad was my hero. My strength. My best friend. It was so surreal that he was lying still and wouldn't breathe!! I was out of my mind with grief. It is still difficult to accept that he's not here. This was surely my worst nightmare.

Now remember, that was the weekend he was going to tell Mom she had Alzheimer's, right? Great Easter. Here we were making funeral plans instead of eating Dad's famous green bean casserole. Following this tragedy, we began the long process of dealing with Mom's progressive illness. She went through all the awful stages of this disease and it certainly took its toll on us. She stayed alone in her home for about six months, and then my sister Karen moved in with her. Later they got a different house together. Not being able to visit the home I grew up in was so sad. Her health and speech worsened, so we eventually moved her into an Alzheimer's care facility. After breaking her hip, as often happens with the elderly, she was moved to a nursing home to get better care.

Mom and I were also the best of buds. We would shop, go to lunch, and talk forever about anything. When I was a teen and on into college, she would party with me and my best friends. We would all go out to lunch, have cocktails, and go to movies. She also played tennis with my boyfriend and best buddy. When I was in grade school she was the bowling coach and Brownie Leader. What a wonderful, graceful, fun, and silly woman. She was the greatest grandma and babysitter, too. My daughter was also very close to both of them, and wrote stories of her hero, her grandpa. She spent a lot of time with them, especially sleepovers on Saturday. Mom would play balloon toss, Memory, and Candyland, and watch movies with her. After church, the three of them went to Pizza Hut or Chop Stix for Chinese buffet. Why did bad things happen to good people? My parents were wonderful servants for the Lord. Why did they have to suffer? Why did *we* have to? Adding to my sadness, my awesome minister died about two months after Dad's funeral, so I could not go to him for grief counseling. I felt so lost.

Larry decided that to get better employment, he needed to get an MBA, so off to the university he went. Unbeknownst to him, he would wake up one day in excruciating, unexplainable pain throughout his entire body. It was a Sunday. To the emergency room we went, only to find out he had viral spinal meningitis. It took three male nurses to hold him down and administer morphine to calm him some. Afterwards they told me they gave him the same amount they would have given a horse. He was so strong, he kept fighting it. The doctor said that the illness would have killed a weaker man. There was no cure, only hope. He spent two weeks in the hospital in the dark. Light was too painful. Was someone watching over him? Was he meant to survive for some greater purpose? I wondered...

While he was in school, I was temporarily supporting the three of us, but he worked some odd jobs to help make ends meet. I had this great career for 14 years and felt very secure. He would tell me, "If you ever lose your job, we are **so** screwed." Well guess what? I lost my job. And yes, we *were* screwed, but not forever. Every time life sent me a challenge, there was always something better waiting for me. They say when one door closes, God opens a window. Remember I figured I was blessed, right? I had several jobs after my long tenure, never making the same income. But I always stayed positive somehow. I know it was due to my faith that God would never give me more than I could handle. It came very close though, many times. Talk about hitting the bottom and crawling back up to ground level. You learn to be patient, frugal, and creative when you don't have money coming in consistently.

It was now the fall of 2005. After my many crummy jobs, we decided to go out on faith – as they call it – and took out a Small Business Administration loan to buy a franchise--an adorable one-of-a-kind specialty bath and body shop. We thought we had the perfect location, the perfect product, and the shop was the perfect size and layout. Larry crafted a 64-page masterpiece of a business plan. Every possible scenario was anticipated except the unimaginable – a catastrophic illness. I had no idea what was coming down the pike that would wreck my dream of being a store owner.

Seven weeks after opening my doors, I was struck down with enormous head pain. I was misdiagnosed a year earlier when I found two small lumps at the base of my neck. I was told I had a couple of sebaceous cysts, and not to worry since I had no pain. So I didn't. I would do a Schwarzenegger impression and jokingly say, "It is not a tumah" and shrug it off. Now it's January of '06, and I had a new, larger lump on the side of my neck about the size of a computer mouse. This time there WAS pain. It wrapped around the base of my neck and across my forehead as if a vise was literally crushing my skull. Talk about seeing stars! On a scale of 1-10, my pain was in the 20s!

I went to a different doctor who told me they were NOT sebaceous cysts, and that I needed a biopsy to find out what I had. Since I had just opened my store, I didn't have any insurance; and knew a biopsy would cost a lot. She said to take some antibiotics to ease the pain, and to check back in five days to pursue other options. Three days went by and I woke up practically paralyzed! My entire body was locked up. I equated it to the Tin Man without his oil can. Imagine every single bone in your body covered in shin splints and then broken, and every single muscle pulled. I couldn't move any part of my body without excruciating pain. Unbearable, wrenching pain with no fluid movement and I had no idea why I hurt. I needed assistance to roll over, get up, lie down, walk, dress, eat, and drink. The only thing I did myself was wipe my own butt! Even then I had to be helped to sit down and get up off the pot. How humiliating.

I stayed in this horrendous pain for two months while attempting to find a company to insure me.

What a dope! No one would touch me. After several mad dashes to the emergency room at 2 a.m. for pain shots, I finally gave up and decided to get the biopsy. At this point if we had to sell everything we owned to get me well, we didn't care. I could not live in this condition any longer. Ever had a neck biopsy? Not pleasant. No anesthesia. They just stuck a long needle in my neck lump and shoved it in and out while sucking out fluid. This continued in a fan-like pattern while they covered the entire area which took about 20 minutes. I squeezed Larry's hand till it turned purple while tears poured down my cheeks. It was horrible! I felt everything. If that wasn't awful enough, they then ran a long camera tube down my nose to my stomach to check for GERD (gastroesophageal reflux disease). I guess I wasn't uncomfortable enough already! I practically crawled out of there; wiped out and pale. I mean, one day I am just fine, the next I am writhing in pain and had to be in a wheelchair if I wanted to go further than 30 feet. Why was this happening to me? What was wrong? Just kill me, please. Put me out of my misery.

My little shop was already suffering as I was never there to promote it. My sister Janice quit her better paying job to manage it for me, and Angela dropped out of college to work there. It was so hard for me not to be there…EVER. I was so weak, and the unknown was making me nuts. The biopsy was March 10. The next evening, the surgeon called to tell us I had cancer. Some kind of lymphoma. My husband answered the phone and my daughter and I overheard the conversation. She called my sisters sobbing her little heart out telling them, "My mom has cancer!"If you have ever heard those words, "YOU HAVE CANCER," then you know exactly how I felt. I was sure it was my arthritis back with a vengeance. *No way* I had cancer! That happened to other people. It was not in the family genes so it had to be a mistake. There was a great urgency in his voice, as he said I was to undergo surgery the next week, and would start treatment the following week. I had to get my house in order now! Larry ran outside, pounded his fists on the ground and screamed. He looked up at the sky yelling "Give it to me, not her. I don't care if I die!"

They say denial is a good thing to help you get through severe issues. I was laughing and talking about wearing wigs with a new cool hairstyle and color. I was all excited about "at least I will finally lose some poundage!" My three sisters would look at each other and whisper, "Oooh, I don't want to be around her when the other shoe drops!!" Denial. It wasn't until I was on the computer a few days later, and a message regarding a certain type of lymphoma popped up. I decided to read it, but wish I hadn't. It went on about the mortality rate of a particular lymphoma. It finally hit me. I COULD DIE! I would lose all my hair! I ran around sobbing inconsolably. I was out of control, racked with fear, and hysterical about what was coming.

Luckily, I did not have that particular lymphoma, but I *did* have a rare one. It made up 5% of the non-Hodgkin's lymphomas. Mantel Cell. The treatment was as aggressive as the cancer itself. I would be in the hospital five days straight every month for treatments, and 2-3 days each week for plasma, platelets, fluids, or antibiotics. If I had a temperature of 102, I had to rush back to stay another five or more days. I got several infections during treatments and had to be put in a "clean" room. Nobody could come in without a mask and gloves. Something else that was odd to me was that my spleen was the size of a football! Apparently the normal size is about that of a baseball. Meanwhile, my home was stripped of all carpeting and redone with wood floors. A bathtub/shower was replaced as it had a small amount of mold. Anything that could collect dust was taken down, packed up, or thrown out. I was pretty much the "girl in a bubble."

Before I could be admitted to the hospital, I had to go through some tests. They had to rush them so I could start Chemo quickly. So one day I have a colonoscopy (where you drink all that gross salty green fluid), the next day a bariatric x-ray (where you have to drink all that gaggy chalky crap) and the next day a bone marrow exam. I was awake lying on my stomach; while a nurse inserted a large 12' syringe into my lower back. She asked me to tell her each time she hit a nerve so she could stop and manipulate the needle around the nerve somehow. Hitting nerves all the way down was pretty rough, and I had to stay perfectly still. She finally hit bottom, pulled out the marrow and the mile long needle, only to tell me she had to do it again to the left side! I did not know I could take more pain, but was fascinated by the procedure, so concentrated on that while asking questions the whole time. I even wanted to look at the marrow afterwards. I told myself if I educated myself about my cancer, was compliant with medications, and then maybe it would be easier to accept.

My first treatment was frightening. Marilyn was with me and things were going fine until the nurse gave me "Cocktail A" (Cocktail B would come the following month). Within seconds, my body was a foot off the bed shaking violently. I threw up like in the *Exorcist* and screamed, "I'm freezing. I'm freezing!" Three nurses came running in and laid several warm blankets over me and then laid on top of me to try and calm me down. My teeth almost shattered right out of my mouth. I locked my eyes on my sister as if to say "No way can I go through this for eight months. I won't survive it!" They adjusted the dosage and I was able to handle it from then on. I flinched each time I returned expecting to fly off the bed again. What a scare!

My entire lymph system was filled with cancer. Pretty eerie seeing that on a PET scan. One week each month I was neutropenic – which meant I had no white blood cells. With no antibodies to fight off infection, I had to be completely protected and not be in public or even go outside. Any germs could potentially kill me during that week. I also had to keep all my critters away from me which was tough, as cuddling them was my greatest form of therapy. That was so frustrating, as it usually hit on the week I wanted to do something out and about, but could only rest. Wednesdays and Saturdays were the days I spent running around with Marilyn. Even on a good day, I had no energy to last more than an hour, if that. She missed the "old" me - full of life and laughter.

I did not know I had stage 4 cancer. As you may already know, it doesn't get any worse than that, hence **there IS no stage 5**! My husband swore all the doctors, nurses, family members and friends to secrecy. He was afraid I would give up if I knew. To this day, I wonder how I would have felt if I *did* know. I stayed "up" for my family as they were falling apart around me. , I remained positive and only went down the "poor me" road once or twice. I am certain my strength came from God because I had always been the "why me" type, and yet *that* Linda never surfaced. Others around me found strength and were encouraged due to MY attitude. How about that!

Speaking of how about that…my awesome husband was at my side every single day during my battle. Having lost his dear mother to cancer, he was frightened history would repeat itself. This is the part when I mentioned earlier about me not knowing how much he really loved me, until I was sick. I never knew how ill I was. I never knew he talked constantly with the doctors and cried with my sisters, and that they did not know from one day to the next if I would pull through. I was unaware that Angela was asking him, "Is Mom gonna die?" How scary for them. I was in such a haze. I knew nothing. I did not find all this out till much later when I asked Larry questions about what went on while I was sick.

My doctor also told me that if my body did not react to the chemo cocktail created for this particular cancer, I would not have made it. She would know from the PET scan, after the first treatment, whether or not the ongoing sessions would be of any consequence. I was scheduled for eight grueling treatments, plus all the in-between visits. I was in the hospital more than I was home. *Hated it!!*

When I *was* home, I often had to sleep on the couch since I was just too weak to make it up the stairs to bed. I had a PIC line in my arm that ran from my upper arm to right above my heart. This was yanked out and replaced four times during my treatment due to an infection or a blood clot in the lines. Not a good thing to happen, as I could have died from either of those things. My poor arms looked like an addict's. Plus they were sore. I had to wrap the area with Saran Wrap if I wanted to shower. There were two openings (ports) at the end of the PIC line. These port tubes came out of my arm and dangled down about four inches – past my elbow. I wrapped that section with a gauze sleeve to cover the ends in an attempt to keep them clean.

My husband and daughter flushed out the two ports with saline solution twice a day to prevent another possible infection. It was a special bond having her treat me, as I knew she was scared. At one point, Larry had to administer shots in my belly twice a day for a week. This procedure was done to prevent more blood clots (which would kill me). That freaked him out and his hands would sweat and shake each time. I promised him he was not hurting me. I didn't want to upset him any more than he already was. Another week he had to hook me up to bags of some fluids to keep me alive and prevent some other disaster from happening that would kill me – I don't even remember. It was either teach him to do it at home or I stay in the hospital another week. I told my doctor Larry could handle it. I wanted to go home. I often cried from boredom, as I missed my home, my bed, my critters, and most of all my family. If I wasn't sleeping, the chemicals kept me very agitated and jumpy, so my attention span was short and I had difficulty doing anything for more than a few minutes; such as crosswords, watching TV, reading, etc.

Losing my hair was harder to deal with than the cancer itself. A woman's hair and lashes are such a huge part of her vanity and identity. It started two weeks after my first treatment. I was taking a shower and while washing my hair, clumps of it came out in my hands. I was mortified! Home alone and totally freaking out, I silently got out of the tub, wrapped up my remaining wet hair, and left the medium-size mass in the tub to show my husband. I took him in there later, pulled back the curtain and said, "It's starting." I sobbed in his big strong arms. I was under the impression that I would not start to lose it for several months. This was the beginning of many more changes that followed.

When I returned for my second visit, my hair was really thinning, so I wore a hairnet to bed in an attempt to keep my pillow free of loose hair. It was early April, and my sister Karen came up on her birthday to cut my hair really short. *That* looked special. It did not help, as I was losing it faster than the net could contain it. The next morning I went down to the hospital salon and had the gal give me a basic military buzz. That still was not working, so my wonderful spouse brought in his razor kit and carefully shaved my head. It was a very somber moment. We looked in the mirror and quietly sobbed. I had four wigs, but never wore them. No matter what, they still looked like doll hair to me, so I wore cute hats and scarves instead. I would paint on my eyebrows to express my mood that day and really missed my long lashes, as my eyes have always been my best asset. Karen came to see me each treatment and brought me an arrangement of silk flowers. I loved fresh flowers but was not allowed to have them as apparently they would make me sicker, if that were even possible. I looked forward to them each visit. Poor Janice worked my store all the time so was not able to leave and visit me in the hospital, but I loved her popping over when I was home. Angela and Marilyn would come down and eat meals with me, but I could tell Angela was uneasy being there. She liked hospitals as much as I did.

In the cancer ward, people were dying around me too often to wrap my head around. I would walk as much as I could in an attempt to keep up my strength. Dragging several bags of meds with me, I would wander up and down my floor. I remember this one girl whose room was packed full of cards, flowers, stuffed animals, ribbons, pictures…the whole room was like an eclectic art gallery. I was not able to tell how old she was, as being bald messes up your perceived age. On my next trip in for the five-day stay, I gathered up the courage to go talk to her, you know, as a fellow cancer sister. I could not locate her room. I thought I was on the wrong floor or corridor. After asking my nurse about her, I was told that she died. I went silent. She said that the girl was never going home, that she had been living the rest of her life in that room on the 6th floor. I stood in the doorway of that once overflowing mass of affection-covered walls, only to see the sterile emptiness awaiting the next guest. That hit too close to home. I was scared. That could be me. I wanted to stay knocked out, as I hated to be there. The drugs made me antsy, food tasted like old pennies, I peed all the time or had diarrhea, and had five or six different chemicals running through my veins at the same time. Oh, let's not forget about being hairless all over. THAT was attractive!

Apparently all the crap I was experiencing wasn't enough, so somehow I developed a compressed disk in my lower back during my third treatment, and was in constant pain. They made a back brace for me to wear when I was up and around attempting to walk. So now I am weak, sick from the drugs, bald, gray, *and* I have relentless back pain. Getting my PET scans was rough as I had to lie on my back on a flat surface for 25 minutes. It would take two people to help me get up due to the extreme back pain. What a hassle! I was in that thing for several months.

August of 2006 was a pivotal time for me. I was released from treatments two months earlier than planned, and sent home for three months without any in-between visits. I didn't know what to do with myself. No more strict routines to follow. I could just hang out. That was strange for me, as I had not been home for more than two days in a row.

Soon I gained strength, and sadly… weight. After finally losing 35 pounds, I was creeping back up once again. Food finally tasted good, and I had an appetite all of a sudden. Wait…I need to digress for a moment. You may have heard the sayings, *Be careful what you wish for* or *Be specific about what you pray for*? Well, I mention this because during my battle with weight gain after getting married, the tubes being tied, and then a few years later a total hysterectomy…I would pray for help with weight loss. I would often say, "Whatever it takes, Lord, whatever it takes to lose my fatness!" Should have been a bit more specific, as the next thing I knew, I had cancer (OK, this was probably just a mere coincidence, but it makes for a good story!).

During my convalescence period at home, I got severely depressed. I went to my doctor in tears and asked her how I could possibly be sad? I was alive, damn it! I beat stage 4 cancer! I should be reveling in my victory! But instead I was missing something. I was not happy and did not know why. I asked her, "Is it possible I feel neglected?" For seven months I was waited on constantly. People came by the house and the hospital to visit. Cards in the mail each week. My husband at my beck and call every minute. Now that I was strong enough to be on my own, all of that stopped. Maybe I didn't like being ok. I must have missed all the attention, therefore making me depressed. She said I was suffering from post traumatic stress disorder (PTSD). That my body had been in a war, and now the war was over and I did not know how to react to the change and the calmness. Made sense, actually.

By October, I had just enough strength to return to my store. As an owner, 10 months away from a new retail shop in a new center is NOT a good thing. By this time, bills were piling up, taxes were not paid, payroll was off the chart, and the very thought-out business plan was pretty much in the

Dumpster. Rent was now due, as were loan payments and franchise fees. Not to mention inventory – I had to have something to sell, right? I was overwhelmed by all of it. Too much was spent on advertising over the prior 10 months and I was starting to feel the pressure of ownership. I witnessed the money slowly being sucked out of the account, like the life that was sucked out of my body for so long.

Even with the increasing bills, business was steady. I had a one-of-a-kind product in an inviting storefront. The quality was next to none, but it was a bit pricey. By the third year, the economy was changing drastically. Gas went up to over $4/gallon, and even my regular customers stayed away. People only had so much disposable income. Do they pay the utilities, buy groceries, or spend $20 on a bottle of custom-made lotion. They were obviously going to Walmart (I know *I* was!).

Sadly, I had no choice but to close up shop, sell off all the products and furnishings, and file bankruptcy. What a blow. My dream was dead. My world was crashing. What now? I had to bring in money to live. As it was, I barely took a salary from the store, but I couldn't go without income for very long. So now I had to deal with being a loser once more. This time I was going from a prominent business owner back to being an employee – working for THE MAN. The status of my previous position was great. I thought I was big time, I guess. My vanity made it difficult for me to humble myself and be among the masses of working folks. As an owner, I came and went as I pleased. No clock punching. I had it made.

I needed to realize that maybe that was MY plan for my life, but not God's. Perhaps He had something else mapped out for me down the road. I bucked up and starting job hunting yet again. If there were ever a position offered for a professional interviewer, I would have gotten it. I would send out maybe three resumes, get two calls, have two interviews, and be offered one or both jobs over the phone as I was driving out of the parking lot, or the next day. They all said I was great in an interview. I responded that I was only being myself; I didn't put on airs, be too bold or too laid-back…just me. Therefore, I was offered *and took* many jobs after closing the store. Too many. I couldn't find what I really wanted to do.

While still searching for that perfect occupation, I returned to many of my former network groups. Some of the sales jobs I had could benefit from these meetings. People were so happy to see me again, as I had pretty much dropped off the face of the earth while ill. I would tell them about my journey when asked, and they would all tell me what an inspiration I was. I remember often while working in my shop with do-rags on my bald little head, customers would tell me the same thing. I had several articles written about my struggle and was featured in some local magazines. By this time, my cancer journey was becoming a blur, and I did not want to be connected to it anymore. That did not make me who I was. I never thought about it until I was asked to repeat my story. After all, my hair had grown back enough to pitch the sweaty head coverings, so why did people want to talk about it? Whenever I did talk about all that I went through, it seemed dreamlike to me. As if it was never really happened. Is that weird?

To this day, if I tell some new person about my journey, I relive each moment as if it were happening at that very second. I can feel the pain of my somewhat paralyzed body, and the extreme pressure in my calves that felt like they would explode if I stood up for more than 20 seconds. The incredible lack of energy, as if any moment I would take my very last breath. My family telling me now how gray my color was and how they never knew if I was going to pull through. It was at that very minute I knew I was saved for a reason.

When I returned to the cancer center for checkups, I would occasionally run into some of the nurses that spent the six months with me. They would hug me and tear up saying they did not think I was going to make it. I was shocked! Again, I never knew I had stage 4 or that I knocked on death's door…twice. I guess I never thought about dying for some reason. I just thought about living. Maybe that is why I am here today. I focused on living. I wanted to get back in the groove, go back to work, pet my seven critters, love on my family, and sleep in my own bed. I just wanted to move on. I was even awarded Franchisee of the Year while in the hospital! I was always in contact with the company attempting to run my store from my hospital bed, checking on ads, products and sales. I refused to give up and give in.

After I was released, I went to some cancer survivor meetings or discussions off and on, and met some people that were very bitter. The narrator would ask us about our journey, and some would still be angry – even after they were many months into remission. They were so mad that cancer had gotten them, and couldn't move past it. I would stand up and say, "I am sorry you are still so bitter. You are alive! Be happy with that! I was blessed for having cancer" The looks I got! I continued by saying how it had made me a better person; that I was more tolerant of diseased, handicapped, or mentally challenged people. That I understood what it was like to have a debilitating or terminal illness. I GOT IT. You truly have to walk in these shoes to understand what we go through. I meet cancer patients and survivors often now, and there truly is an unspeakable bond between us.

I landed a new sales job in February of 2010. I was back! My colleagues told me, "Wow – you look great! You are your old self again! It is so good to see you with passion about what you do! You have found your calling!" I felt good. I was having fun selling, networking, and just being me.

I started wondering if I survived to inspire people somehow. Was my purpose on earth to help others go through this battle? If so, how would I do that? What did I know about anything? These thoughts still run through my mind. I had the strongest urge from "somewhere" to write this all down. Was God prompting me to put in words something that may help someone else be ok while going through cancer? Is the message that it doesn't matter who you are or where you came from, that anyone can get it, and anyone can get through it?

I may never know the real reason I wrote this book. Only that I will continue to try to inspire those I meet, with or without illnesses; and to continue focusing on living life to the fullest. I was given a second chance to do something worthwhile with my remaining days.

I wait patiently for the message...